Comprehensive Guide to Cardiac and Respiratory Emergencies

Advanced Diagnostic and Management Strategies

Carter D. Ball, MD, FACC

© 2024 Carter D. Ball, MD, FACC. All rights reserved.

No part of this book may be reproduced, distributed, or transmitted in any form or by any means, including photocopying, recording, or other electronic or mechanical methods, without the prior written permission of the publisher, except in the case of brief quotations for critical reviews or articles.

Acknowledgements

I would like to express my sincere gratitude to all those who contributed to the completion of this book. First and foremost, I am deeply thankful to my family for their unwavering support and patience throughout this endeavor. I am also indebted to my esteemed colleagues and mentors, whose expertise, insights, and constructive feedback have been integral to the development of this work. Special thanks to the medical professionals and researchers whose contributions to the fields of cardiology and respiratory medicine continue to shape and advance clinical practice.

I would also like to acknowledge the editorial and publishing teams for their exceptional professionalism and dedication in bringing this book to life. Lastly, my deepest appreciation goes to my patients, whose experiences have continually inspired my commitment to advancing knowledge and improving care in the fields of cardiac and respiratory emergencies.

Without the collective support of these individuals, this work would not have been possible.

Carter D. Ball, MD, FACC

Preface

Cardiac and respiratory emergencies represent some of the most critical situations in clinical medicine, requiring prompt diagnosis, accurate interpretation, and timely intervention to optimize patient outcomes. In an era of rapid advancements in medical technology and evolving therapeutic strategies, healthcare professionals must be equipped with the knowledge and skills necessary to navigate the complexities of these emergencies effectively.

"Comprehensive Guide to Cardiac and Respiratory Emergencies: Advanced Diagnostic and Management Strategies" is designed to serve as an essential resource for clinicians, providing in-depth insights into the latest diagnostic techniques, management approaches, and evidence-based practices. This guide is particularly valuable for medical students, residents, emergency physicians, cardiologists, pulmonologists, and other healthcare providers working in acute care settings.

The book begins by addressing the fundamental concepts of emergency medicine, detailing essential diagnostic tools and techniques, including advanced cardiac imaging, spirometry, pulmonary function tests, and the interpretation of electrocardiograms (ECGs). A central focus is placed on the integration of these diagnostic modalities with clinical decision-making, ensuring that healthcare providers can make timely and accurate assessments of critically ill patients.

The chapters are structured to guide clinicians through a variety of life-threatening conditions, from acute coronary syndromes and myocardial infarctions to respiratory failure, pulmonary embolism, and chronic obstructive pulmonary disease (COPD). Each chapter is thoroughly researched and reflects the latest evidence in clinical practice, incorporating not only common conditions but also rare and complex cases that healthcare providers may encounter in the emergency setting.

Key diagnostic challenges are addressed through the use of clinical scenarios, diagnostic algorithms, and step-by-step management strategies, allowing for a hands-on approach that enhances practical skills. The book also places significant emphasis on decision-making under pressure, offering guidance on when and how to escalate care, from non-invasive techniques to advanced interventions such as mechanical ventilation, invasive monitoring, and surgical management.

In addition to core diagnostic and therapeutic approaches, this book delves into the broader context of cardiac and respiratory care, including the management of comorbidities, secondary prevention strategies, and long-term follow-up considerations. The integration of multidisciplinary perspectives ensures a holistic approach to patient care, emphasizing collaboration between different specialties and healthcare providers.

This guide is not merely a theoretical exploration of acute conditions; it is a comprehensive, hands-on manual that prioritizes patient-centered care and seeks to improve clinical outcomes through evidence-based practices. The chapters are presented in a clear, structured format, facilitating both rapid reference and deep study.

As the landscape of medical care continues to evolve, so too must the skills of healthcare professionals. "Comprehensive Guide to Cardiac and Respiratory Emergencies" provides the tools necessary to meet the demands of modern emergency medicine, ensuring that clinicians are not only prepared to respond to acute crises but are also equipped with the expertise to navigate the increasingly complex world of cardiac and respiratory emergencies.

By the time you finish this guide, you will be better equipped to diagnose, manage, and treat patients in crisis, offering the highest standard of care and making a meaningful difference in the lives of those affected by life-threatening cardiac and respiratory conditions.

Carter D. Ball, MD, FACC
2024

Acknowledgement
Preface
List of Abbreviations

Table of Contents

Chapter 1: Acute Coronary Syndrome: A Practical Guide to Diagnosis and Management

1.1 Introduction
1.2 Classification of Acute Coronary Syndrome (ACS)
1.3 Angina Pectoris and Unstable Angina
1.4 Atypical Presentations (Angina Equivalents)
1.5 Clinical Examination in ACS
1.6 ECG Diagnostic Criteria for STEMI, NSTEMI, and Posterior Wall MI
1.7 Sgarbossa Criteria for STEMI in LBBB
1.8 Wellens' Syndrome and T Wave Abnormalities
1.9 Diagnostic Insights from Lead aVR

1.10 Cardiac Enzyme Testing in ACS
1.11 STEMI and NSTEMI Management Protocols
1.12 Risk Stratification: TIMI Score

Chapter 2: Hypertensive Crisis Management

2.1 Introduction to Hypertensive Crisis
2.2 Hypertensive Emergency and Urgency
2.3 Clinical Assessment and Patient Presentation
2.4 Diagnostic Investigations for Hypertensive Crisis
2.5 Management Strategies: General Principles
2.6 Specific Conditions Requiring Urgent Management
2.7 Blood Pressure Reduction Goals and Intravenous Medications

Chapter 3: Diagnostic Approaches in Cardiology

3.1 Overview of Diagnostic Modalities
3.2 Role of Echocardiography

3.3 Advanced Imaging Techniques (CT, MRI, PET)
3.4 Blood Biomarkers and Their Diagnostic Significance
3.5 Diagnostic Pathways for Common Cardiac Conditions

Chapter 4: Cardiac Emergencies and Their Management

4.1 Acute Heart Failure and Pulmonary Edema
4.2 Arrhythmias: Diagnosis and Urgent Management
4.3 Pericarditis and Cardiac Tamponade
4.4 Acute Aortic Dissection
4.5 Cardiogenic Shock: Clinical Features and Management

Chapter 5: Pharmacological Management in Cardiology

5.1 Antiplatelet and Anticoagulant Therapy
5.2 Beta-Blockers, ACE Inhibitors, and ARBs
5.3 Nitrates and Calcium Channel Blockers

5.4 Statins and Lipid-Lowering Therapies
5.5 Emergency Drug Protocols in Acute Cardiac Conditions

Chapter 6: Paroxysmal Supraventricular Tachycardia (PSVT)

1. Introduction
1.1 Definition and Mechanisms of PSVT
1.2 Types of PSVT (AVNRT, AVRT, Atrial/Sinoatrial Reentrant Tachycardia)

2. Management
2.1 Acute Intervention for Unstable Patients
2.2 Vagal Maneuvers for Stable Patients

3. Electrocardiographic Characteristics
3.1 Heart Rate and Rhythm
3.2 QRS Duration and P Waves

4. Procedural Techniques
4.1 Carotid Massage: Procedure, Risks, and Contraindications

4.2 Adenosine Administration: Dosing, Pharmacokinetics, and Contraindications

5. Adjunct and Alternative Treatments
5.1 Magnesium Sulfate and Calcium Channel Blockers
5.2 Radiofrequency Ablation for Recurrent PSVT

Chapter 7: Wide Complex Tachycardias (WCT)

1. Introduction
1.1 Definition and Classification
1.2 Common Causes: Ventricular vs. Supraventricular Origins

2. Ventricular Tachycardia (VT)
2.1 Monomorphic VT: Sustained vs. Nonsustained
2.2 Polymorphic VT and Torsades de Pointes

3. Ventricular Fibrillation (VF)

3.1 ECG Characteristics
3.2 Pathophysiology

4. Management
4.1 Unstable VT: Synchronized Cardioversion
4.2 Stable VT: Medications and Cardioversion
4.3 Torsades de Pointes: Magnesium and Amiodarone

5. Summary of Electrical Energy Dosage

Chapter 8: Valvular Emergencies

1. Introduction
1.1 Native Valve vs. Prosthetic Valve Emergencies

2. Native Valve Emergencies
2.1 Acute Aortic Regurgitation: Causes and Features
2.2 Acute Mitral Regurgitation: Causes and Features

3. Investigations
3.1 Key Diagnostic Tests
3.2 Role of Imaging and Blood Tests

4. Management of Regurgitant Lesions
4.1 Cardiogenic Shock and Heart Failure
4.2 Definitive Surgical Interventions

5. Prosthetic Valve Emergencies
5.1 Valvular Thrombosis: Risk Factors and Clinical Features
5.2 Acute Obstructive Valve Thrombus: Diagnosis and Treatment

Chapter 9: Cardiomyopathy in Emergencies

1. Introduction
1.1 Types of Cardiomyopathy
1.2 Pathophysiology of Emergency Presentations

2. Hypertrophic Cardiomyopathy
2.1 Clinical Features and Diagnosis

2.2 Management of Acute Symptoms

3. Dilated Cardiomyopathy
3.1 Causes and Presentation
3.2 Emergency Management

4. Restrictive Cardiomyopathy
4.1 Clinical Features and Diagnostic Approach
4.2 Acute Treatment Strategies

5. Takotsubo Cardiomyopathy
5.1 Pathophysiology and ECG Findings
5.2 Management and Prognosis

Chapter 10: Pericardial Emergencies

1. Introduction
1.1 Overview of Pericardial Disorders
1.2 Classification of Pericardial Emergencies

2. Acute Pericarditis
2.1 Causes and Clinical Features
2.2 ECG Changes and Management

3. Pericardial Effusion
3.1 Etiology and Clinical Presentation
3.2 Echocardiographic Evaluation

4. Cardiac Tamponade
4.1 Pathophysiology and Hemodynamic Impact
4.2 Emergency Management: Pericardiocentesis

5. Constrictive Pericarditis
5.1 Diagnosis and Differentiation from Tamponade
5.2 Surgical and Medical Interventions

Chapter 11: Chronic Obstructive Pulmonary Disease (COPD)

1. Introduction
1.1 Overview of COPD and Subtypes
1.2 Diagnostic Criteria: Spirometry Findings

2. Pulmonary Function Tests (PFTs)
2.1 Spirometry
2.2 Additional Tests: CBC, Creatinine, Electrolytes, CXR, ECG, ABG

3. Management of Acute Exacerbation of COPD
3.1 Initial Steps: ABC Assessment and Oxygen Therapy
3.2 Treatment of Bronchospasm: Nebulization, Steroids, Magnesium Sulfate
3.3 Antibiotic Use
3.4 Non-Invasive Ventilation (NIV): Indications and Benefits
3.5 Mechanical Ventilation: Indications

4. Discharge Recommendations
4.1 Correct MDI Technique via Spacer
4.2 Prescribed Maintenance Medications

5. Spirometry and Lung Volumes
5.1 Differentiation of Lung Diseases
5.2 Overview of Lung Volumes and Capacities

Chapter 12: Pulmonary Embolism (PE)

1. Introduction
1.1 Pathophysiology of Pulmonary Embolism
1.2 Risk Factors and Predisposing Conditions

2. Clinical Presentation
2.1 Symptoms and Signs
2.2 Differential Diagnosis

3. Diagnostic Approach
3.1 Wells Score and Risk Stratification
3.2 Imaging Modalities: CT Pulmonary Angiography, Doppler Ultrasound
3.3 Laboratory Tests: D-dimer, ABG

4. Management of Pulmonary Embolism
4.1 Initial Stabilization: ABC Approach
4.2 Anticoagulation Therapy
4.3 Thrombolysis: Indications and Contraindications
4.4 Surgical and Catheter-based Interventions

5. Long-term Management and Follow-up
5.1 Secondary Prevention Strategies
5.2 Risk Stratification for Recurrent PE

6. Special Considerations
6.1 Pregnancy and Pulmonary Embolism
6.2 PE in Cancer Patients

Chapter 13: Pneumothorax

1. Introduction
1.1 Definition and Classification
1.2 Pathophysiology of Pneumothorax

2. Types of Pneumothorax
2.1 Primary Spontaneous Pneumothorax
2.2 Secondary Spontaneous Pneumothorax
2.3 Traumatic Pneumothorax
2.4 Iatrogenic Pneumothorax

3. Clinical Features and Diagnosis

3.1 Symptoms and Physical Examination Findings
3.2 Diagnostic Imaging: Chest X-ray, Ultrasound, CT Scan

4. Management
4.1 Initial Stabilization: ABC Approach
4.2 Observation and Oxygen Therapy
4.3 Needle Aspiration and Chest Tube Insertion
4.4 Surgical Intervention: Indications

5. Complications and Follow-up
5.1 Recurrent Pneumothorax
5.2 Long-term Monitoring

Chapter 14: Respiratory Failure

1. Introduction
1.1 Definition and Types of Respiratory Failure
1.2 Pathophysiology and Etiology

2. Acute vs Chronic Respiratory Failure
2.1 Distinguishing Features

2.2 Common Causes

3. Clinical Assessment
3.1 Symptoms and Signs
3.2 Diagnostic Workup: ABG, Imaging, Pulmonary Function Tests

4. Management of Respiratory Failure
4.1 Oxygen Therapy: Nasal Cannula, Venturi Mask, High-flow Oxygen
4.2 Non-Invasive Ventilation (NIV): CPAP and BiPAP
4.3 Invasive Mechanical Ventilation: Indications and Strategies
4.4 Pharmacological Management

5. Specific Considerations
5.1 ARDS (Acute Respiratory Distress Syndrome)
5.2 COPD Exacerbation and Respiratory Failure
5.3 Neuromuscular Causes of Respiratory Failure

6. Long-term Management and Rehabilitation

6.1 Weaning Strategies
6.2 Pulmonary Rehabilitation Programs
6.3 Monitoring and Follow-up

List of Abbreviations

A&E – Accident and Emergency
ABG – Arterial Blood Gas
ACLS – Advanced Cardiovascular Life Support
ARDS – Acute Respiratory Distress Syndrome
ASA – American Society of Anesthesiologists
AST – Aspartate Aminotransferase
BLS – Basic Life Support
CABG – Coronary Artery Bypass Grafting
CCU – Coronary Care Unit
COPD – Chronic Obstructive Pulmonary Disease
CPR – Cardiopulmonary Resuscitation
CT – Computed Tomography
ECG – Electrocardiogram
ED – Emergency Department
EMS – Emergency Medical Services
ETCO2 – End-Tidal Carbon Dioxide

FIO2 – Fraction of Inspired Oxygen
HR – Heart Rate
ICU – Intensive Care Unit
IPAP – Inspiratory Positive Airway Pressure
IV – Intravenous
LBBB – Left Bundle Branch Block
LDL – Low-Density Lipoprotein
MI – Myocardial Infarction
MVA – Motor Vehicle Accident
NIV – Non-Invasive Ventilation
PE – Pulmonary Embolism
PFT – Pulmonary Function Test
PCI – Percutaneous Coronary Intervention
PEEP – Positive End-Expiratory Pressure
PTCA – Percutaneous Transluminal Coronary Angioplasty
RV – Right Ventricle
SARS – Severe Acute Respiratory Syndrome
SPO2 – Oxygen Saturation
TAA – Thoracic Aortic Aneurysm
TBI – Traumatic Brain Injury
VF – Ventricular Fibrillation
VT – Ventricular Tachycardia
WBC – White Blood Cell

Chapter 1
Acute Coronary Syndrome: A Practical Guide to Diagnosis and Management

Introduction

Acute Coronary Syndrome (ACS) encompasses a spectrum of clinical conditions characterized by myocardial ischemia and infarction. ACS is classified into three main categories based on clinical presentation and ECG findings:

1. ST-Elevation Myocardial Infarction (STEMI)

2. Non-ST-Elevation Myocardial Infarction (NSTEMI)

3. Unstable Angina (UA)

Angina Pectoris

Angina pectoris presents as:

Substernal discomfort triggered by exertion

Radiation of pain to the shoulder, jaw, or inner arm

Relief within 10 minutes of rest or nitroglycerin.

Unstable Angina

Key features include:

Resting angina lasting over 20 minutes

New-onset angina limiting physical activity significantly

Increasing frequency, duration, or decreased exertion threshold compared to prior angina episodes.

Atypical Presentations (Angina Equivalents)

Patients, especially those with diabetes, may exhibit symptoms other than chest pain, such as:

Breathlessness

Epigastric pain accompanied by vomiting

Palpitations

Presyncope or syncope.

Examination

Physical findings suggestive of ACS include:

Signs of hypoperfusion: cold extremities, hypotension, altered mental status, sweating

Features of cardiac failure.

ECG Diagnostic Criteria

STEMI

ST elevation: New elevation at the J point in two anatomically contiguous leads. Diagnostic thresholds:

≥1 mm in all leads except V2 and V3

In V2 and V3:

≥1.5 mm in women

≥2 mm in men over 40 years

≥2.5 mm in men under 40 years.

NSTEMI/UA

Horizontal or down-sloping ST depression ≥0.5 mm in two contiguous leads.

T-wave inversion ≥1 mm in two contiguous leads with prominent R waves (R/S ratio >1).

Old Myocardial Infarction (MI)

Absence of left ventricular hypertrophy (LVH) or left bundle branch block (LBBB) is necessary. Key findings include:

Q waves ≥0.03 seconds and ≥1 mm deep in two contiguous leads

QS complexes in two contiguous leads.

Posterior Wall MI

Typically associated with inferior or lateral infarctions, posterior MI indicates a higher risk of left ventricular dysfunction. Isolated posterior MI requires urgent coronary reperfusion.

ECG findings in posterior leads (V7–V9):

ST elevation ≥0.5 mm

Q waves.

Changes in anterior leads (V1–V3) suggesting posterior MI:

Horizontal ST depression

Tall, broad R waves (>30 ms)

Upright T waves

Dominant R wave (R/S ratio >1).

Posterior Lead Placement

V7: Left posterior axillary line at the same horizontal plane as V6.

V8: Left scapular tip in line with V6.

V9: Left paraspinal region at the same horizontal plane as V6.

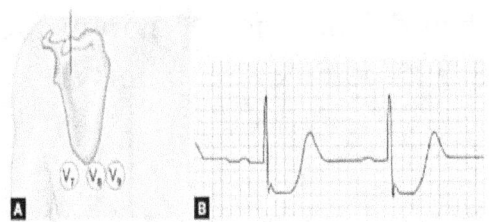

Fig. 1A & 1B: (A) Posterior Lead Placement; (B) Anterior Lead ECG Changes in Posterior Wall MI

Sgarbossa Criteria for Diagnosing STEMI in the Presence of LBBB

The Sgarbossa criteria are a diagnostic tool to identify STEMI in patients with a left bundle branch block (LBBB). The three components of the criteria and their scoring are:

1. Concordant ST elevation ≥1 mm in a lead with a positive QRS complex – 5 points

2. ST depression ≥1 mm in leads V1, V2, or V3 – 3 points

3. Discordant ST elevation ≥5 mm in a lead with a negative QRS complex – 2 points

A score of ≥3 points indicates a 90% specificity and 36% sensitivity for diagnosing STEMI. Sensitivity improves with serial or previous ECG comparisons.

Wellens' Syndrome

Wellens' syndrome is characterized by specific T wave abnormalities in leads V2–V3, indicating a critically stenotic proximal left anterior descending (LAD) artery. This condition is highly specific for impending extensive anterior wall myocardial infarction (MI).

Key Features:

T wave changes: Deeply inverted or biphasic T waves in V2–V3.

Patients are often pain-free or asymptomatic during ECG recording.

Cardiac enzymes: May show mild elevation.

Risk: High likelihood of anterior wall MI within days to weeks.

Patterns of T Wave Abnormalities:

1. Type A (Biphasic T Waves): Initial positivity followed by terminal negativity (25% of cases, Fig. 2A).

2. Type B (Deeply Inverted T Waves): Symmetrical and deep T wave inversion (75% of cases, Fig. 2B).

Evolution: T waves often progress from Type A to Type B over time.

Understanding these criteria ensures early recognition and management of these high-risk conditions, potentially preventing adverse cardiac outcomes.

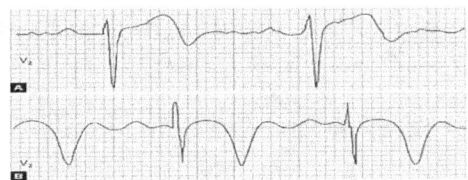

Fig. 2A & 2B: Wellens' Syndrome - Type A (Biphasic T Waves) and Type B (Deep T Wave Inversion)

Lead aVR: Key Insights and Diagnostic Importance

Lead aVR, often overlooked, provides critical information about the right ventricular outflow tract (RVOT) and basal septum. Its significance becomes evident in acute coronary syndromes (ACS), particularly in diagnosing left main coronary artery (LMCA) occlusion.

Key ECG Findings in aVR During LMCA Occlusion:

ST elevation ≥1 mm in lead aVR.

ST elevation in aVR greater than in lead V1.

Horizontal ST depression in leads I, II, and V4–V6.

Cardiac Enzyme Testing in ACS

Appropriate cardiac enzyme testing enhances diagnostic accuracy for ACS:

1. Single acute chest pain episode: Send Troponin T.

2. Recent chest pain with worsening angina (within 1 week): Send Troponin T and CK-MB.

3. NSTEMI/Unstable Angina (UA): Repeat Troponin T within 3–6 hours of the initial test.

STEMI Management

Timely diagnosis and intervention are vital—"time is myocardium." Delays in management can result in irreversible myocardial damage.

Initial Approach:

1. ECG Monitoring:

Up to 45% of initial ECGs may be nondiagnostic.

Repeat ECGs every 10 minutes for suspected ongoing ischemia.

2. Aspirin: Administer 300 mg stat without delay.

3. Oxygen Therapy: Only if SpO_2 <94%, targeting 94–98%.

Pain Management:

Nitrates:

Sublingual nitroglycerin 0.4 mg every 5 minutes (up to three doses).

Persistent pain: Start GTN infusion at 5 µg/min, titrate while monitoring BP. Contraindicated in inferior wall MI (IWMI) or if SBP <90 mmHg.

Morphine:

3–5 mg IV stat, repeated after 15 minutes if pain persists. Persistent pain indicates ongoing ischemia.

Medication Protocol:

Antiplatelets:

Aspirin 325 mg non-enteric coated (chewed).

Clopidogrel: 300 mg PO loading dose (<75 years) or 75 mg PO (>75 years).

Statins: Atorvastatin 80 mg stat.

Beta-Blockers: Metoprolol 25 mg PO if no contraindications (avoid heart failure, COPD, or AV block).

Anticoagulation Therapy:

For Primary PCI:

Unfractionated heparin: 70 U/kg bolus (max 5,000 U).

For Thrombolysis or No PCI:

Unfractionated heparin: 100 U/kg bolus followed by infusion to maintain aPTT 1.5 -- 2.5× normal.

Enoxaparin: 30 mg IV bolus + 1 mg/kg SC every 12 hours.

Reperfusion Strategies:

Primary PCI: Preferred within 12–24 hours of symptom onset.

Thrombolysis: For <12 hours post-onset if PCI is unavailable. May extend to 24 hours in symptomatic patients.

Streptokinase: 1.5 million U IV over 60 minutes.

Tenecteplase: 30–50 mg IV bolus.

NSTEMI Management

Initial Steps:

Evaluate Airway, Breathing, Circulation (ABC).

Administer oxygen if SpO_2 <94% (target 94–98%).

Pain Management:

Nitrates: Same as STEMI protocol.

Morphine: 3–5 mg IV, repeat after 30 minutes if necessary.

Medications:

Antiplatelets: Same as STEMI.

Anticoagulation:

Unfractionated heparin: 5,000 U IV stat, then q6h.

Enoxaparin: 1 mg/kg SC q12h (adjust for renal impairment).

Beta-Blockers: Same as STEMI.

Key Considerations:

Avoid thrombolysis in NSTEMI.

Monitor high-risk patients using the TIMI score to guide intervention timing.

TIMI Score: Prognostication for UA/NSTEMI

The Thrombolysis in Myocardial Infarction (TIMI) score helps estimate the risk of adverse events within 14 days.

Risk Factor	Points
Age > or = 65 years	1
> or = 3 coronary risk Factors (e g., HTN, DM, smoking)	1
Prior coronary stenosis > or = 50%	1
ST - Segment deviation on admission ECG	1
> or = Aegina episode in 24 hours	1
Elevated cardiac biomarkers	1
Aspirin use in the past 7 days	1

Interpretation:

0–2 points: Low risk (4–7% event rate).

3–4 points: Intermediate risk (8.3–19.9%).

5–7 points: High risk (26.2–40.9%).

Timely monitoring and intervention based on TIMI scores improve outcomes in ACS patients.

Chapter 2
Hypertensive Crisis Management

Hypertensive Emergency

Hypertensive emergencies are characterized by severe hypertension, typically with a diastolic blood pressure (DBP) exceeding 120 mm Hg, accompanied by signs of acute end-organ damage. This condition demands immediate medical intervention to mitigate the risk of fatal outcomes. Blood pressure (BP) reduction should occur within minutes to hours to stabilize the patient.

Hypertensive Urgency

In hypertensive urgency, DBP also exceeds 120 mm Hg, but there is no evidence of acute end-organ damage. Unlike a hypertensive emergency, immediate BP reduction is not necessary, and treatment can proceed over hours to days without risk of complications.

Clinical Assessment

Patient Presentation:

Hypertensive crises may occur in individuals with or without pre-existing chronic hypertension.

Assess for end-organ damage signs, such as:

Projectile vomiting.

Focal neurological deficits.

Peripheral pulse irregularities.

Chest pain.

Pulmonary edema or papilledema.

History:

Obtain a thorough medication history, focusing on compliance.

Note that sudden discontinuation of antihypertensive medications can trigger rebound hypertension.

Diagnostic Investigations

1. Electrocardiogram (ECG):

Assess for left ventricular hypertrophy (LVH) or acute coronary syndrome (ACS).

2. Chest X-ray:

Look for pulmonary edema.

3. Urinalysis:

Identify signs of acute glomerulonephritis, such as casts or active sediment.

4. Serum Studies:

Evaluate serum electrolytes and creatinine levels.

5. Cardiac Enzymes:

Measure if ACS is suspected.

6. Brain Imaging (CT/MRI):

Perform for neurological symptoms, hypertensive retinopathy, or nausea/vomiting.

7. Contrast-Enhanced CT/MRI or Transesophageal Echocardiography:

Use if an aortic dissection is suspected.

Management Strategies

General Principles

Initiate antihypertensive therapy promptly upon diagnosing uncontrolled hypertension.

For hypertensive urgency, aim for a gradual reduction of BP over 24 hours with oral medications.

For hypertensive emergencies, prioritize intravenous (IV) medications to enable precise BP control.

Specific Conditions

1. Acute Aortic Dissection:

Rapid BP reduction to lower aortic shearing forces.

2. Hemorrhagic Stroke with High BP:

Target systolic BP (SBP) between 140–160 mm Hg.

Management of Hypertensive Emergency

Blood Pressure Reduction Goals:

Lower mean arterial pressure (MAP) by 10–20% in the first hour and approximately 15% over 24 hours.

For aortic dissection, reduce MAP by 25% in the first hour and another 25% within 24 hours.

Calculation of MAP:

$$MAP = DBP + 1/3 (SBP - DBP)$$

Intravenous Medications:

Nitroglycerin: 5–100 μg/min infusion; monitor BP every 10 minutes.

Labetalol: Initial 20 mg IV bolus; repeat doses every 10 minutes up to 300 mg (contraindicated in heart failure and COPD).

Esmolol: Loading dose of 250–500 μg/kg over 1 minute, followed by infusion (avoid heart failure and COPD).

Special Considerations:

Avoid using beta-blockers alone in pheochromocytoma due to unopposed alpha-adrenergic activation.

Oral Transition Medications:

Add agents like amlodipine, nifedipine, metoprolol, losartan, or hydrochlorothiazide while tapering IV drugs.

Monitoring:

Observe patients for at least 12 hours.

Discharge on two oral antihypertensives if BP stabilizes.

Management of Hypertensive Urgency

Blood Pressure Reduction Goals:

Decrease MAP by 25–30%, or achieve an SBP <160 mm Hg or DBP <100 mm Hg within 24 hours.

Medication Protocol:

In previously treated hypertensives:

Restart prior antihypertensives in noncompliant patients.

Adjust dosages or add diuretics.

For new diagnoses:

Start with agents like nifedipine, metoprolol, losartan, prazosin, or hydrochlorothiazide.

Reassess BP after 4 hours; add additional agents as needed.

Monitoring and Follow-up:

Initiate two medications in cases of extremely high BP (>200/120 mm Hg).

Discharge stable patients with advice to follow up in an outpatient setting.

Emergencies Requiring Special Attention

Effective management of hypertensive crises depends on early recognition, appropriate pharmacological intervention, and meticulous monitoring of BP trends and end-organ function.

Chapter 3
Pulmonary Edema

Introduction

Pulmonary edema is a frequent and potentially life-threatening condition that presents as acute respiratory distress. Immediate and continuous cardiac monitoring is essential for affected patients. The term "flash pulmonary edema" refers to a sudden, severe onset of decompensated heart failure caused by a rapid increase in left ventricular (LV) diastolic pressure, leading to swift accumulation of fluid within the pulmonary interstitial and alveolar spaces.

Causes

1. Cardiogenic

Left ventricular failure

Mitral stenosis

2. Noncardiogenic

Pneumonia

Inhaled toxins

Aspiration

Acute radiation pneumonitis

Hypoalbuminemia

3. Idiopathic or Incompletely Understood

High-altitude pulmonary edema

Neurogenic pulmonary edema

Narcotic overdose

Post-cardioversion

Investigations
Key diagnostic tests include:

Complete blood count (CBC)

Serum electrolytes, creatinine, and urea levels

Troponin T to assess myocardial injury

Electrocardiogram (ECG) for cardiac abnormalities

Chest X-ray (CXR) to evaluate pulmonary congestion

Arterial blood gas (ABG) analysis to assess oxygenation and acid-base status

Management

1. Initial Stabilization

Position the patient upright to alleviate respiratory distress.

Administer oxygen therapy with a high concentration (60–100%) via a face mask, aiming for SpO2 levels of 94–98%.

2. Hemodynamically Unstable Arrhythmias

Perform urgent synchronized cardioversion if required.

3. Diuretics

Administer furosemide (40–120 mg IV) or torsemide (20–60 mg IV), ensuring SBP >100 mm Hg prior to administration.

4. Management of Acute Coronary Syndrome (ACS)

Initiate heparin and antiplatelet therapy if indicated.

For SBP >90 mm Hg, provide sublingual glyceryl trinitrate (GTN) 5 mg or a spray.

Start GTN infusion at 5–10 μg/min, titrating the dose every 15–20 minutes to target a MAP around 70 mm Hg.

5. Cardiogenic Shock

For SBP <90 mm Hg, use noradrenaline (0.1 -- 0.5 μg/kg/min) or dopamine (5–20 μg/kg/min) infusion.

6. Renal Considerations

Consider dialysis in cases of oliguric renal failure, rising creatinine, or lack of response to diuretics within 4 hours.

7. Respiratory Support

Initiate continuous positive airway pressure (CPAP) for severe Type 1 respiratory failure, starting with FiO2 100% and PEEP at 5 cm H2O.

Transition to invasive ventilation if clinical deterioration occurs.

High-Altitude Pulmonary Edema (HAPE)

Overview
HAPE occurs in unacclimatized individuals at altitudes above 2,000 meters, especially during physical exertion. While commonly seen in tourists and mountaineers, this noncardiogenic pulmonary edema can be fatal. Symptoms include dyspnea, dry cough, headache, and reduced exercise tolerance. Hypoxia plays a central role in its pathophysiology.

Related Conditions

Acute Mountain Sickness (AMS): Nausea, vomiting, and headache.

High-Altitude Cerebral Edema (HACE): Symptoms include ataxia, confusion, and coma, which may coexist with HAPE.

Management

1. Immediate descent to lower altitudes is critical.

2. For mild AMS, administer acetazolamide 125–250 mg orally twice daily to expedite acclimatization.

3. Provide supplemental oxygen (2–4 L/min) to maintain SpO2 >90%.

4. If oxygen is unavailable, prescribe nifedipine 10 mg orally every 4–6 hours for HAPE.

5. For severe HACE or HAPE, administer dexamethasone 4 mg orally or IV as a loading dose, followed by 4 mg every 6 hours.

6. Prophylactic use of inhaled β2-agonists such as salmeterol may reduce the incidence of HAPE.

Chapter 4
Atrial Fibrillation (AF)

Introduction

Atrial fibrillation (AF) is a common cardiac arrhythmia frequently encountered in emergency departments. It is defined by an irregularly irregular pulse and requires management tailored to the duration and underlying cause of the condition.

Clinical Presentation

AF may manifest with symptoms such as palpitations, chest pain, breathlessness, fainting, low blood pressure, or embolic events like stroke or peripheral embolism. Its classification helps guide treatment:

1. Paroxysmal AF: Resolves spontaneously or with intervention within seven days.

2. Persistent AF: Persists for more than seven days without self-termination.

3. Long-term Persistent AF: Continues for over 12 months.

4. Permanent AF: Chronic AF where rhythm control measures are either unsuccessful or not pursued.

Electrocardiographic (ECG) Characteristics

Typical findings in AF include:

Atrial rates around 300 beats per minute.

An irregularly irregular rhythm.

Absence of P waves, replaced by fibrillation waves.

Causes

AF can result from various cardiac and non-cardiac conditions, including:

Cardiac causes: Rheumatic or ischemic heart disease, hypertension, heart failure, cardiomyopathy, or pericarditis.

Non-cardiac causes: Thyrotoxicosis, electrolyte disturbances (e.g., low potassium or magnesium), or substance use such as alcohol and stimulants.

Investigations

Diagnostic evaluation typically includes:

Blood tests: Complete blood count, electrolyte levels, renal function, magnesium, and thyroid function tests.

Imaging: Chest X-rays to assess underlying pulmonary or cardiac conditions.

Cardiac biomarkers and drug levels when clinically indicated.

Management

1. Initial Stabilization

Ensure airway, breathing, and circulation are stable.

Address electrolyte imbalances and correct metabolic acidosis, if present.

2. Rate and Rhythm Control

Unstable Patients
For patients with hypotension, acute heart failure, or other signs of instability, synchronized cardioversion is recommended, starting at 50

Joules and increasing as needed. Adequate sedation should be administered. Avoid cardioversion in chronic AF or conditions like severe mitral stenosis or left ventricular dysfunction due to embolic risk. If initial attempts fail, amiodarone infusion and correction of electrolyte abnormalities should follow.

Stable Patients
In hemodynamically stable individuals, pharmacologic rate control is prioritized. Common options include beta-blockers (e.g., metoprolol), calcium channel blockers (e.g., diltiazem, verapamil), or digoxin in selected cases. Amiodarone may also be considered for persistent or chronic cases.

3. Anticoagulation

Patients with rheumatic AF require anticoagulation to prevent thromboembolic events.

For non-rheumatic AF, anticoagulation is guided by a structured risk assessment. In patients with a higher stroke risk, oral anticoagulants like warfarin are recommended, while low-risk patients may not require therapy.

Anticoagulation is essential before and after cardioversion in chronic cases to prevent clot-related complications.

Evidence-Based Practice

Research highlights the importance of tailored risk assessment in managing AF. Using clinical tools to evaluate stroke and thromboembolic risks ensures effective and safe anticoagulation, minimizing complications while improving patient outcomes.

By following these guidelines, clinicians can approach AF management with confidence, ensuring both symptom control and the prevention of long-term complications.

Chapter 5
Atrial Flutter

Introduction

Atrial flutter is a cardiac arrhythmia characterized by rapid and regular atrial depolarization, typically at a rate of approximately 300 beats per minute (bpm). The ventricular response, influenced by atrioventricular (AV) conduction, is commonly regular and occurs at about 150 bpm due to a 2:1 AV conduction ratio.

Clinical Manifestations

Patients with atrial flutter often present with symptoms such as palpitations, fatigue, lightheadedness, and shortness of breath. Other manifestations may include chest discomfort, low blood pressure, anxiety, near-fainting episodes, or, less commonly, syncope. These symptoms result from the heart's inability to pump efficiently during episodes of rapid atrial activity.

Electrocardiogram (ECG) Characteristics

Key diagnostic features of atrial flutter on an ECG include:

Atrial rate: Typically around 300 bpm.

Absence of typical P waves: Instead, atrial activity appears as a saw-tooth pattern, also known as F waves, most evident in leads II, III, and aVF.

AV conduction: Usually exhibits a 2:1 ratio, leading to a ventricular rate that is half of the atrial rate, provided there is no underlying AV node dysfunction.

Evidence-Based Analysis

The regular pattern and rapid rate of atrial flutter contribute to hemodynamic instability in some cases, particularly when the ventricular rate exceeds 150 bpm. This rhythm disturbance is closely associated with underlying heart disease and may predispose individuals to thromboembolic events, particularly stroke. Accurate diagnosis using ECG findings and timely intervention are essential for improving patient outcomes and minimizing complications.

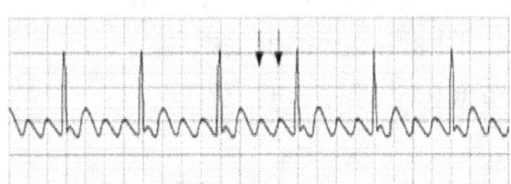

Fig. 3: Atrial Flutter with 4:1 AV Conduction

Management of Atrial Flutter

Stable Patients

For hemodynamically stable patients, administer amiodarone at an initial dose of 5 mg/kg in 5% dextrose over 30 minutes, followed by 10 mg/kg infused over 23 hours. The management priorities are similar to those in atrial fibrillation and include:

1. Rate Control: Achieved using the same protocols as in atrial fibrillation.

2. Restoration of Sinus Rhythm: This can be done pharmacologically or through radiofrequency ablation.

3. Embolism Prevention: Employ anticoagulation strategies identical to those used in atrial fibrillation.

Unstable Patients

For patients presenting with unstable rhythms, such as hypotension, signs of shock, altered mental status, ischemic chest pain, or acute heart failure:

Perform synchronized cardioversion starting at 50 J, increasing to 100 J and then 200 J if necessary.

Ensure adequate sedation using midazolam (2 mg IV) or ketamine (1–2 mg/kg IV) to maintain patient comfort.

This approach addresses both symptom control and the underlying risk of thromboembolism effectively.

Chapter 6
Paroxysmal Supraventricular Tachycardia (PSVT)

Introduction

Paroxysmal supraventricular tachycardia (PSVT) refers to sudden-onset and self-terminating supraventricular tachycardias (SVTs) that exclude atrial fibrillation (AF), atrial flutter, and multifocal atrial tachycardia (MAT). PSVTs commonly arise from reentry mechanisms, with variations in the site of reentry.

The primary causes include:

1. Atrioventricular nodal reentrant tachycardia (AVNRT): ~60%

2. Atrioventricular reentrant/reciprocating tachycardia (AVRT): ~30%

3. Atrial or sinoatrial nodal reentrant tachycardia: ~10%

Management

Acute intervention aims to stabilize the patient and manage the arrhythmia effectively.

1. For Unstable Patients:

Indicators of instability include hypotension, shock, altered mental status, ischemic chest pain, or acute heart failure.

Initiate synchronized cardioversion starting at 25 J, escalating to 100 J and 150 J if needed. Ensure proper sedation with midazolam (2 mg IV) or ketamine (1–2 mg/kg IV) to maintain patient comfort.

2. For Stable Patients:

Employ vagal maneuvers, such as breath-holding or the Valsalva maneuver, to reduce AV node conduction and potentially disrupt the reentrant circuit.

Electrocardiographic Characteristics

Heart Rate: Greater than 100 bpm

Rhythm: Regular

P Waves: Typically absent

QRS Duration: Less than 0.12 ms

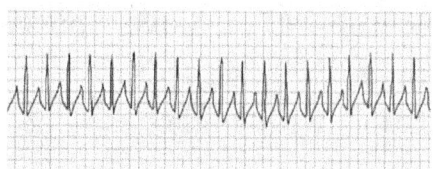

Fig. 4: ECG Representation of Paroxysmal Supraventricular Tachycardia.

Carotid Massage

Carotid massage involves applying external pressure to the carotid sinus, which activates baroreceptors to stimulate vagal activity and suppress sympathetic output. This results in a transient reduction in sinoatrial (SA) node activity and atrioventricular (AV) node conduction. The procedure is performed by applying firm pressure to the carotid sinus, typically located below the angle of the mandible at the thyroid cartilage level, for 5–10 seconds. If ineffective, it can be repeated on the opposite side after a 1–2 minute interval. While generally safe, potential risks include hypotension, bradycardia, transient ischemic attack (TIA), stroke, or arrhythmias. Carotid massage is contraindicated if a carotid bruit is detected.

Adenosine Administration

Adenosine, a purine nucleoside, significantly slows heart rate and prolongs AV nodal conduction. It is delivered via rapid intravenous (IV) bolus over 1–2 seconds, followed by a saline flush to ensure rapid transit to the heart. Administration should occur in a supine patient under continuous electrocardiogram (ECG) and blood pressure (BP) monitoring.

Dosing:

Initial adult dose: 6 mg (100 μg/kg in children).

If ineffective, administer 12 mg (200 μg/kg in children) after 1–2 minutes.

A third dose of 12 mg (300 μg/kg in children) can be given after another 1–2 minutes if needed.

For central IV administration, the initial dose should not exceed 3 mg.

Pharmacokinetics: Adenosine's half-life is 10–20 seconds due to rapid intracellular metabolism, necessitating a saline flush post-administration.

Contraindications: Sinus node dysfunction, second- or third-degree AV block, long QT syndrome, hypotension, and conditions like asthma or chronic obstructive pulmonary disease (COPD).

Side Effects: Common adverse effects include flushing, chest discomfort, dyspnea, metallic taste, and a sensation of impending doom.

Adjunct and Alternative Treatments

Magnesium sulfate (2 g IV over 5–10 minutes) may address deficiencies and treat arrhythmias.

Calcium channel blockers (e.g., verapamil, diltiazem) and beta-blockers (e.g., metoprolol, esmolol) serve as alternatives for acute supraventricular tachycardia (SVT) management.

For recurrent paroxysmal supraventricular tachycardia (PSVT), radiofrequency ablation is recommended, offering high success rates.

Chapter 7
Wide Complex Tachycardias (WCT)

Introduction

Wide complex tachycardias (WCT) are fast heart rhythms, typically exceeding 100 beats per minute, and are characterized by a QRS duration greater than 0.12 seconds. These arrhythmias are commonly linked with ischemic heart disease or acute myocardial infarction, and they include conditions such as ventricular tachycardia (VT) and ventricular fibrillation (VF). While WCT usually originates from the ventricles, a supraventricular tachycardia (SVT) can also present as WCT if there is a conduction abnormality or aberrancy.

Ventricular Tachycardia (VT)

VT is categorized into monomorphic and polymorphic forms:

Monomorphic VT: This form of VT features regular QRS complexes at a rate between 150–200 beats per minute. It is further divided into:

Sustained VT: Lasts longer than 30 seconds or causes hemodynamic instability.

Non-sustained VT: Occurs with more than three beats but lasts less than 30 seconds.

Polymorphic VT: In this type, the QRS complexes vary in shape and size within the same lead. A specific variant of polymorphic VT, Torsades de Pointes, is characterized by a changing axis of the QRS complexes, swinging from positive to negative directions. This arrhythmia is often triggered by drugs that prolong the QT interval, such as quinidine, procainamide, and tricyclic antidepressants.

Ventricular Fibrillation (VF)

VF is marked by complete disorganization of the depolarization and contraction of the ventricular myocardium. On an ECG, it presents as a fine or coarse zigzag pattern with no identifiable P waves or QRS complexes. VF results in the absence of pulse and blood pressure, making it a critical emergency.

Management

1. Unstable Ventricular Tachycardia (e.g., hypotension, shock, altered mental state, ischemic chest pain, or acute heart failure):

Synchronized cardioversion should be initiated, starting at 100 J, and increasing to 150 J and then 200 J if necessary. Sedation, using agents like midazolam or ketamine, is required for patient comfort.

2. Stable Ventricular Tachycardia:

For monomorphic VT, if the rhythm is regular and monomorphic, adenosine should be given as a 6 mg IV bolus, followed by a second dose of 12 mg if needed.

If there is no response to adenosine, amiodarone (150 mg over 10 minutes, followed by 1 mg/min for 6 hours), magnesium sulfate (2 g IV over 3–5 minutes), or lidocaine (100 mg IV push) can be administered.

If medications fail, synchronized cardioversion at 100 J should be performed with appropriate sedation.

For polymorphic VT with long QT (Torsades de Pointes), the treatment includes magnesium sulfate (2 g IV), followed by amiodarone (150 mg over 10 minutes) and possibly lidocaine (1–1.5 mg/kg IV) if the condition persists.

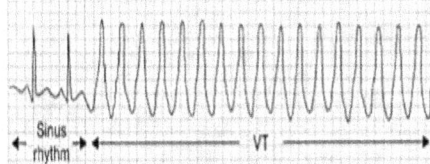

Fig. 5: Ventricular tachycardia.

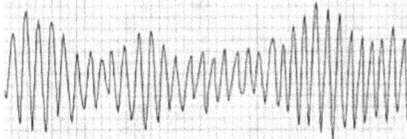

Fig. 6: Torsades de pointes.

If the previous medications are ineffective, unsynchronized cardioversion should be administered at 200 J, along with appropriate sedation (e.g., midazolam 2 mg IV or ketamine 1–2 mg/kg IV). In cases where the arrhythmia remains refractory, additional treatments such as beta blockers, calcium channel blockers, or phenytoin may be considered.

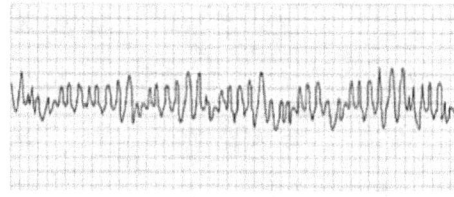

Fig. 7: Ventricular fibrillation.

Ventricular Fibrillation (VF)

For ventricular fibrillation, the Advanced Cardiovascular Life Support (ACLS) protocol should be followed for cardiac arrest management. This includes defibrillation at 200 J, with amiodarone administered as a 300 mg IV bolus after the third shock, in accordance with ACLS guidelines.

Summary of Electrical Energy Dosage for Cardioversion

The choice of energy levels for cardioversion varies depending on the arrhythmia type and waveform characteristics. For narrow complex rhythms such as supraventricular tachycardia (SVT) or atrial flutter, synchronized cardioversion is performed with an initial dose of 50–100 J. In cases of atrial fibrillation (AF), which is irregular in rhythm, the recommended energy for monophasic defibrillators starts at 200 J, while biphasic defibrillators typically require 120–200 J.

For wide complex tachycardias that are regular, such as ventricular tachycardia (VT), synchronized cardioversion should begin with 100 J. However, if the rhythm is irregular, such as in ventricular fibrillation (VF), unsynchronized defibrillation is necessary. Monophasic devices require 360 J, whereas biphasic devices generally need 200 J for optimal outcomes.

The type of rhythm (regular vs. irregular) and waveform (narrow vs. wide complex) guide the selection of energy levels and the synchronization mode. Synchronized cardioversion is used for rhythms with identifiable R waves, while unsynchronized defibrillation is reserved for disorganized rhythms like VF. These principles ensure effective and safe rhythm management.

Chapter 8
Valvular Emergencies

Introduction

Valvular emergencies are critical conditions that can be broadly categorized into two types:

1. Native valve emergencies

2. Prosthetic valve emergencies

Native Valve Emergencies

Acute native valve emergencies predominantly involve regurgitation. However, patients with inadequately treated chronic mitral stenosis (MS) may present with exacerbation of congestive heart failure.

Acute Aortic Regurgitation

Causes:
Infective endocarditis, rupture of the sinus of Valsalva, or aortic dissection involving the aortic root.

Clinical Features:
Symptoms of cardiac failure, a pronounced pulmonary component of the second heart sound (P2), and a left ventricular (LV) third heart sound (S3). Notably, cardiomegaly is absent.

Acute Mitral Regurgitation

Causes:
Chordae tendineae rupture, papillary muscle rupture, acute endocarditis, or blunt chest trauma.

Clinical Features:

Presents with pulmonary edema, hypotension, and LV S3. Similar to acute aortic regurgitation, cardiomegaly is not present.

Investigations

Key diagnostic tests include:

Electrocardiogram (ECG)

Echocardiography (ECHO)

Chest X-ray

Cardiac enzymes to exclude acute coronary syndrome (ACS)

Blood tests, including electrolytes, creatinine, and complete blood count (CBC).

Management of Regurgitant Lesions

Address cardiogenic shock and heart failure promptly.

For acute mitral regurgitation, use an intra-aortic balloon pump to reduce aortic impedance and decrease regurgitant volume.

Avoid beta-blockers as they prolong diastole, worsening regurgitation.

Initiate empirical antibiotics for infective endocarditis (IE) if fever and peripheral IE features are present.

Definitive management requires surgical intervention, including valve replacement.

Mitral Stenosis

For mitral stenosis, medical treatment focuses on alleviating symptoms:

Diuretics: Relieve pulmonary congestion.

Atrial Fibrillation Control: Rate control and rhythm management.

Anticoagulation: Prevent arterial embolism in high-risk patients.
Definitive treatment involves mechanical intervention, such as balloon mitral valvotomy (BMV), valve repair, or valve replacement.

Prosthetic Valve Emergencies

Both mechanical and biologic prosthetic valves are susceptible to complications, including paravalvular regurgitation caused by suture failure or dehiscence related to endocarditis. Mechanical prostheses are also at risk for acute stenosis due to pannus formation or thrombosis.

Acute Valvular Thrombus and Embolism

High-Risk Period: Up to three months post-surgery, particularly in noncompliant patients with anticoagulation therapy.

Clinical Features: Stroke or pulmonary embolism may occur.

Treatment: Adjust anticoagulation to achieve a therapeutic international normalized ratio (INR) of 3–4.

Acute Obstructive Valve Thrombus

Causes: Inadequate anticoagulation leading to subtherapeutic levels.

Clinical Presentation: Gradual or sudden onset of dyspnea, fatigue, and possible embolic events. Absence of prosthetic valve clicks upon auscultation is a significant indicator of prosthetic valve stenosis or occlusion.

Diagnosis: Urgent echocardiography to measure gradients across the prosthetic valve.

Treatment:

Surgical Intervention: Recommended for left-sided prosthetic valves causing severe symptoms (NYHA class III–IV).

Fibrinolytic Therapy: Reserved for recent-onset (less than 14 days) obstructive thrombosis with mild symptoms (NYHA class I–II) and small thrombi (<0.8 cm²).

Emergency surgery is mandatory for large or mobile thrombi (≥0.8 cm²) in left-sided prosthetic valves.

Fibrinolysis is suitable for obstructive thrombosis in right-sided prosthetic valves.

Valve or Paravalvular Regurgitation

Commonly observed during the early postoperative period or as a result of infective endocarditis.

Clinical Features: Changes in prosthetic valve sounds, dyspnea, or heart failure symptoms.

Treatment: Manage heart failure medically, followed by surgical correction.

Conclusion

Acute valvular emergencies require prompt recognition and tailored intervention. Native valve emergencies often necessitate surgery for definitive care, while prosthetic valve complications require careful anticoagulation management or urgent surgical intervention, depending on severity and presentation. Early diagnosis and appropriate treatment can significantly improve patient outcomes.

Chapter 9
Fundamentals of Electrocardiogram (ECG)

Heart Rate Calculation

The method for determining heart rate varies based on rhythm regularity:

Regular Rhythms (Lead II):

Divide 300 by the number of large squares between consecutive R-R intervals.

Alternatively, divide 1,500 by the number of small squares between consecutive R-R intervals.

Irregular Rhythms (Lead II):

Count the number of R waves within 30 large squares, then multiply the result by 10.

Characteristics of Normal Sinus Rhythm

A normal sinus rhythm demonstrates the following features:

A regular rhythm with a heart rate between 60–100 bpm in adults.

Every QRS complex is preceded by a normal P wave.

P waves are upright in leads I and II and inverted in aVR, indicating a normal P wave axis.

The PR interval remains consistent throughout.

The QRS complexes are narrow, measuring less than 100 milliseconds.

Determining the QRS Axis

The axis of the QRS complex is assessed using leads I and aVF by observing whether the deflections are predominantly positive or negative:

Lead I positive, aVF positive: Indicates a normal axis (0° to +90°).

Lead I negative, aVF positive: Suggests right axis deviation (+90° to +180°).

Lead I positive, aVF negative: Indicates left axis deviation (0° to –90°).

Lead I negative, aVF negative: Represents extreme right axis deviation (–90° to +180°).

Key Duration Parameters

Normal ECG parameters include:

P Wave Duration: Less than 120 milliseconds, representing atrial depolarization.

PR Interval: Between 120–200 milliseconds, indicating the time required for the electrical impulse to travel through the AV node.

QRS Complex: Measures 70–100 milliseconds, reflecting ventricular depolarization.

QT Interval: Extends up to 440 milliseconds, representing the time for ventricular depolarization and repolarization.

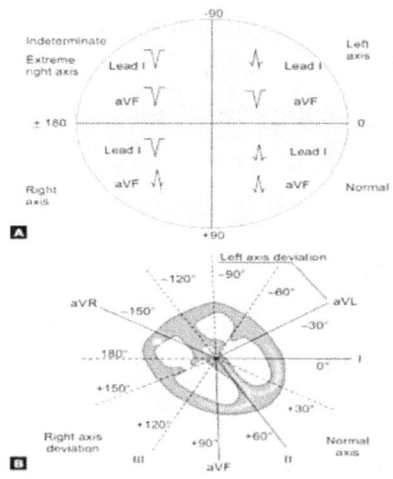

Fig. 8A AND B: (A) Diagram of ECG Axis Deviation; (B) ECG Axis

P Wave:

The P wave, the first positive deflection in the ECG complex, represents atrial depolarization. Normal, P pulmonale, and P mitrale patterns are depicted in Figure 2. A normal P wave has the following characteristics:

Duration: <120 ms (3 small squares)

Amplitude: <2.5 mm in limb leads and <1.5 mm in chest leads

Positive in lead II and negative in lead aVR

P Pulmonale indicates right atrial enlargement, commonly seen in conditions such as COPD, pulmonary hypertension, and tricuspid stenosis. It is characterized by:

P wave amplitude >2.5 mm in inferior leads (II, III, aVF)

P wave amplitude >1.5 mm in leads V1 and V2

P Mitrale suggests left atrial enlargement, typically associated with mitral stenosis, and is characterized by:

P wave duration >120 ms in lead II

Biphasic P wave in lead V1

Q Wave: The Q wave is the first negative deflection in the ECG complex, reflecting left-to-right depolarization of the interventricular septum. Characteristics of a normal Q wave include:

Duration: <40 ms (1 small square)

Amplitude: <2 mm

Depth: <25% of the subsequent R wave's height

Q waves are normal in leads III and aVR. They are pathological if:

Duration >0.04 seconds (1 small square)

Depth >25% of the R wave's amplitude

R Wave: The R wave is the first positive deflection in the QRS complex, indicating depolarization of the ventricular walls. It is the largest deflection in the QRS complex.

S Wave: The S wave is the negative deflection after the R wave, reflecting depolarization of the Purkinje fibers. It is usually a small wave.

T Wave: The T wave represents ventricular repolarization and appears as a positive deflection following the QRS complex. It is upright in most leads, except in aVR and V1. T wave amplitude typically measures:

<5 mm in limb leads

<10 mm in precordial leads

T Wave Abnormalities:

Peaked T waves: Tall, narrow, and symmetrical, commonly seen in hyperkalemia (Figure 3).

Hyperacute T waves: Broad and asymmetrical, often seen in early ST-elevation myocardial infarction (STEMI) (Figure 4).

Left Ventricular Hypertrophy (LVH) Diagnostic Criteria: To diagnose LVH, any of the following voltage criteria must be met:

S wave in V1 + R wave in V5 or V6 >35 mm (Sokolov Lyon criteria)

S wave in V3 + R wave in aVL >28 mm in men or >20 mm in women (Cornell criteria)

R wave in aVL >11 mm

Additional ECG features of LVH may include left atrial enlargement and left axis deviation.

Left Bundle Branch Block (LBBB) Diagnostic Criteria:

Broad QRS complex (>120 ms)

Dominant S wave in lead V1

Monophasic, 'M' shaped R wave in lateral leads (I, aVL, V5, and V6)

Prolonged R wave peak time >60 ms in left precordial leads (V5-V6)

Absence of Q waves in lateral leads (I, V5, V6)

LBBB is typically pathological and can result from ischemic heart disease, anterior wall MI, aortic stenosis, hypertension, dilated cardiomyopathy, hyperkalemia, and digoxin toxicity.

Right Bundle Branch Block (RBBB) Diagnostic Criteria:

Broad QRS complex (>120 ms)

RSR' pattern in leads V1-V3 ('M' shaped QRS complex)

Wide, slurred S wave in lateral leads (I, aVL, V5, V6) RBBB can be a normal finding in healthy young individuals, but it can also indicate pathological causes, including ischemic heart disease, rheumatic heart disease, cor pulmonale, pulmonary embolism, myocarditis, and atrial septal defects.

Brugada Syndrome: Brugada syndrome is a genetic disorder that leads to sudden cardiac arrest in structurally normal hearts. The ECG pattern is characterized by:

Coved ST segment elevation (>2 mm) in leads V1-V3

A negative T wave following the elevation (Brugada sign) (Figure 5)

Syncope and sudden cardiac arrest can be triggered by factors such as fever, hypokalemia, hypothermia, and certain medications (e.g., flecainide, propafenone, beta blockers, calcium channel blockers, nitrates, cocaine, and alcohol). The definitive treatment is implantation of a cardioverter defibrillator (ICD).

Chapter 10
Bronchial Asthma

Introduction

Asthma is a chronic inflammatory disorder characterized by airway hyperresponsiveness, variable airflow obstruction, and reversibility with bronchodilators.

Clinical Features

Asthma presents with recurrent episodes of:

Chest tightness

Breathlessness

Wheezing

Cough

Differentiation between Asthma and Chronic Obstructive Pulmonary Disease (COPD):

A comparison between asthma and COPD is summarized below:

Feature	Asthma	COPD
Age of the Onset	Children/young adults	Older > 40 years
Allergy/Atopy	Common	Rare
Family History	Common	Rare
Smoking Association	Not causal, exacerbates	Strong association (> 10 pack-years)
Chronic sputum production	Rare	Common
Airway inflammations	Eosinophilic	Neutrophilic

Airway Obstruction	Reversible	Minimal/no reversibility
Disease	Stable exacerbations	Progressive worsening with exacerbations
Response to Bronchodilators	Immediate relief as needed	Routine use for symptom control
Response to steroids	Essential for control	Beneficial in moderate/severe cases

Classification of Acute Asthma

1. Life-Threatening Asthma:

Peak expiratory flow rate (PEFR): <33% of best/predicted

SpO_2 <92%, normocapnia

Signs: Silent chest, cyanosis, poor respiratory effort

Complications: Bradycardia, arrhythmias, hypotension, exhaustion, confusion, coma

2. Near-Fatal Asthma:

Raised arterial partial pressure of carbon dioxide ($PaCO_2$)

Requires mechanical ventilation

3. Acute Severe Asthma:

PEFR: 33–50% of best/predicted

Respiratory rate: >25 breaths/min

Pulse rate: >110 beats/min

Unable to complete sentences

4. Moderate Exacerbation:

PEFR: 50–75% of best/predicted

Talks in phrases

Respiratory rate: <25 breaths/min

Pulse rate: <110 beats/min

Differential Diagnosis for Wheezing:
Consider alternative diagnoses, including:

Upper airway obstruction

Foreign body aspiration

Endobronchial malignancy

Pulmonary edema (cardiac asthma)

COPD

Investigations

Diagnostic evaluations include:

Complete blood count (CBC)

Serum creatinine and electrolytes

Chest X-ray

Electrocardiogram

Arterial blood gas (ABG) analysis for moderate/severe cases

Note: ABG is unnecessary for mild asthma cases.

Management of Acute Asthma

1. Immediate Stabilization:

Ensure airway, breathing, and circulation (ABC)

Administer high-flow oxygen (maintain SpO_2 >94%)

2. Pharmacological Therapy:

Steroids: Oral prednisolone (40–50 mg/day) or IV hydrocortisone (200 mg stat, then 100 mg every 6 hours)

Nebulization: Salbutamol (5 mg) + ipratropium bromide (0.5 mg), repeated every 15 minutes (three doses)

For Persistent Symptoms:

Repeat nebulization if severe wheezing persists

Consider IV magnesium sulfate (2 g over 20 minutes) or subcutaneous epinephrine (0.3–0.5 mg)

3. Severe/Refractory Cases:

Initiate non-invasive ventilation to reduce respiratory effort

Do not delay intubation for life-threatening asthma

4. Antibiotics:

Indicated only if infection is evident (fever, purulent sputum)

5. Medications Not Recommended:

Aminophylline infusions are no longer advocated for acute asthma management.

Discharge Recommendations

Prednisolone: 40–50 mg/day for 5–7 days

Maintenance therapy:

Inhaled Steroid + Long-Acting Beta-Agonist (LABA)

Budesonide + formoterol (200 µg, 2 puffs twice daily)

Salmeterol + fluticasone (125–250 µg, 2 puffs twice daily)

Reliever: Salbutamol (100 µg, as needed)

Note: Acute exacerbations during pregnancy require aggressive management to prevent fetal hypoxia. All asthma medications are safe for use in pregnancy.

Key Concept: Peak Expiratory Flow Rate (PEFR)

PEFR measures the maximum exhalation rate during a forced expiratory effort following full inspiration.

Chapter 11
Chronic Obstructive Pulmonary Disease (COPD)

Introduction

Chronic obstructive pulmonary disease (COPD) is a progressive respiratory condition marked by persistent airflow limitation due to chronic inflammation triggered by prolonged exposure to harmful particles or gases. The primary contributors include cigarette smoking and sustained exposure to biomass fuels like firewood. COPD encompasses subtypes such as emphysema, chronic bronchitis, and chronic obstructive asthma, all of which share the common feature of airflow obstruction. Diagnosis is confirmed through spirometry, which demonstrates post-bronchodilator irreversibility.

Chronic Bronchitis: Defined by a productive cough lasting at least three months over two consecutive years, provided other causes of chronic cough (e.g., bronchiectasis) are excluded. Diagnosis is primarily clinical.

Emphysema: Characterized by abnormal and irreversible enlargement of airspaces beyond the terminal bronchioles, accompanied by airspace wall destruction without significant fibrosis.

Pulmonary Function Tests (PFTs)

Spirometry is the cornerstone for evaluating lung function, performed both pre- and post-bronchodilator (e.g., 400 μg albuterol inhalation). COPD is identified by an FEV1/FVC ratio below 70% and a post-bronchodilator FEV1 below 80%. Additional diagnostic tests include:

Complete blood count (CBC)

Creatinine and electrolyte levels

Chest X-ray (CXR)

Electrocardiogram (ECG)

Arterial blood gas (ABG) for assessing moderate-to-severe cases.

Management of Acute Exacerbation of COPD

Management aims to stabilize the patient, alleviate symptoms, and prevent further deterioration.

Initial Steps

1. Airway, Breathing, Circulation (ABC) Assessment: Prioritize securing airway patency and ensuring effective oxygenation.

2. Oxygen Therapy: Administer oxygen to maintain SpO2 between 88-92%. Avoid high-flow oxygen to prevent CO2 retention.

Treatment of Bronchospasm

Nebulization: Combine salbutamol (5 mg) and ipratropium (0.5 mg), administered every 15 minutes for three doses. Use air-driven nebulizers to avoid hyperoxia.

Steroids: Administer IV hydrocortisone (200 mg stat, followed by 100 mg every 6 hours).

Magnesium Sulfate: Consider a single dose of 2 g IV infusion over 20 minutes for refractory bronchospasm.

Terbutaline: Administer 0.25 mg subcutaneously every 20 minutes (up to three doses), or initiate an infusion at 0.05 µg/kg/min in severe cases.

Use of Antibiotics

Initiate antibiotics when infection is evident, such as in patients with fever or purulent sputum. Select antibiotics based on the CURB score.

Non-Invasive Ventilation (NIV)

NIV is the preferred approach for managing type 2 respiratory failure. It reduces intubation rates, mortality, and hospital stays.

Indications for NIV:

Respiratory acidosis: pH < 7.35 and $PaCO_2$ > 45 mm Hg.

Severe dyspnea: Fatigue with accessory muscle use or paradoxical breathing.

Hypoxemia: Persistent despite oxygen therapy.

Mechanical Ventilation

Mechanical ventilation is considered when patients fail or cannot tolerate NIV.

Discharge Recommendations

Verify and teach the correct metered-dose inhaler (MDI) technique using a spacer.

Prescribe maintenance medications:

Inhaled steroids + long-acting β-agonists (e.g., formoterol-budesonide or salmeterol-fluticasone).

Reliever inhaler: Salbutamol 100 µg, as needed.

Proper MDI Technique via Spacer

1. Shake the MDI and attach it to the spacer.

2. Exhale gently to empty the lungs.

3. Place the spacer mouthpiece in the mouth, press the MDI once, and inhale deeply.

4. Hold the breath for 5–10 seconds.

5. Take two additional breaths through the spacer before removing it.

6. Wait one minute and repeat the process for the second puff.

Spirometry and Lung Volumes

Spirometry aids in differentiating obstructive from restrictive lung diseases. Residual lung volumes, not directly measured by spirometry, are assessed via helium dilution or body plethysmography. Key lung volumes and capacities include:

Tidal Volume (TV): Air exchanged during normal breathing (~500 mL in a 70 kg adult).

Inspiratory Reserve Volume (IRV): Additional air inhaled beyond a normal breath (~3,300 mL).

Expiratory Reserve Volume (ERV): Additional air exhaled after a normal exhalation (~1,700 mL).

Residual Volume (RV): Air remaining in lungs after maximal exhalation (~1,800 mL).

Vital Capacity (VC): Total air volume that can be exhaled after maximal inhalation (TV + IRV + ERV, ~5,500 mL).

Total Lung Capacity (TLC): Maximum air volume in the lungs after full inspiration (VC + RV, ~7,500 mL).

Note on Spirometry Use

Spirometry remains vital for assessing and monitoring COPD progression. Proper interpretation of results informs clinical decision-making, ensuring optimal management strategies for each patient.

Chapter 12
Pulmonary Embolism

Introduction

Pulmonary embolism (PE) is an acute and potentially fatal condition caused by a venous thromboembolism that travels to the pulmonary artery or its branches. Most often, the source of these emboli is a thrombus originating in the deep veins of the lower extremities or the pelvic veins. The emboli can obstruct blood flow at the pulmonary artery bifurcation or within smaller lobar branches, leading to significant clinical consequences.

Clinical Presentation

Patients with PE often present with dyspnea, the most common symptom. Other clinical manifestations include pleuritic chest pain, cough, hemoptysis, and signs of deep vein thrombosis (DVT), such as leg swelling and tenderness. Diagnosis requires a high level of suspicion, particularly in patients with risk factors and unexplained hypoxemia.

The modified Wells scoring system is a valuable tool for assessing the likelihood of PE.

Parameters	Points
Clinical symptoms of DVT (e.g., leg swelling tenderness)	3
Other diagnosis less likely than PE	3
Heart rate > 100 beats/min	1.5
Immobilization (> or = 3 days) or recent surgery (4 weeks)	1.5
Previous DVT/PE	1.5

Hemoptysis	1
Malignancy	1

Interpretation:

PE likely: Score > 4.0

PE unlikely: Score ≤ 4.0

Investigations

1. Electrocardiography (ECG):

Most common finding: sinus tachycardia.

The classical S1Q3T3 pattern (S wave in lead I, Q wave in lead III, and inverted T wave in lead III) occurs in only 5–10% of cases.

2. D-dimer Testing:

Elevated D-dimer levels (> 500 ng/mL) suggest thrombus formation but are nonspecific.

A negative D-dimer test has a high negative predictive value, effectively ruling out PE in low-risk patients.

3. Chest X-ray:

Typically normal but may reveal findings such as Westermark's sign (regional oligemia) or Hampton's hump (wedge-shaped opacity).

4. Echocardiography (ECHO):

May show right ventricular (RV) dysfunction in severe cases.

McConnell's sign: RV free-wall hypokinesis with preserved apical motion, a specific finding for PE.

5. CT Pulmonary Angiography (CTPA):

The gold standard for confirming PE.

Look for intraluminal filling defects indicating obstruction.

Management

1. Oxygen Therapy:

Maintain peripheral capillary oxygen saturation (SpO2) > 90%.

2. Intravenous Fluids:

Use cautiously to avoid fluid overload, which can impair RV function.

3. Vasopressors:

Administer norepinephrine for patients in shock.

Consider dobutamine to improve myocardial contractility if needed.

4. Anticoagulation Therapy:

For hemodynamically stable patients:

Start with heparin (5,000 units IV bolus) or enoxaparin (1 mg/kg subcutaneously).

For unstable patients:

Initiate thrombolytic therapy unless contraindicated.

5. Thrombolytic Agents:

Alteplase (tPA): 100 mg IV over 2 hours.

Streptokinase: Initial 250,000 units IV over 30 minutes, followed by 100,000 units/hour for 24 hours.

6. Absolute Contraindications for Thrombolysis:

Prior intracranial hemorrhage.

Known cerebral vascular malformations or malignant neoplasms.

Recent ischemic stroke (< 3 months).

Suspected aortic dissection.

Active bleeding disorders.

Recent major trauma or head injury (< 3 months).

7. Surgical or Catheter-Based Embolectomy:

Considered when thrombolysis is contraindicated or ineffective.

Conclusion

Management of PE requires a timely, systematic approach emphasizing risk stratification, diagnostic precision, and evidence-based interventions. Prompt recognition and treatment, including anticoagulation, thrombolysis, or embolectomy when necessary, significantly improve outcomes in this potentially life-threatening condition.

Chapter 13
Pneumothorax

Types of Pneumothorax

1. Primary Spontaneous Pneumothorax:

Occurs in individuals without known pulmonary disease or those with undiagnosed conditions.

More frequently observed in smokers.

2. Secondary Spontaneous Pneumothorax:

Develops in individuals with underlying lung diseases, such as chronic obstructive pulmonary disease (COPD).

Commonly caused by the rupture of a bleb or bulla.

3. Traumatic Pneumothorax:

A result of blunt or penetrating chest trauma.

Frequently associated with injuries sustained in accidents or physical trauma.

4. Iatrogenic Pneumothorax:

Induced by medical procedures, including:

Transthoracic needle aspiration.

Thoracentesis.

Central venous catheter insertion.

Mechanical ventilation or cardiopulmonary resuscitation (CPR).

Symptoms and Signs

Sudden or gradual onset of dyspnea.

Sharp, pleuritic chest pain, often exacerbated by breathing or coughing.

Diagnosis

1. Chest X-Ray (CXR):

Identifies radiolucent air in the pleural space and the absence of lung markings.

2. Ultrasonography:

Detects the absence of lung sliding, a hallmark of pneumothorax.

Determining the Size of Pneumothorax on CXR:

Small Pneumothorax: A distance of ≤2–3 cm between the collapsed lung and chest wall.

Large Pneumothorax: A rim of air >3 cm.

Management

1. Tension Pneumothorax (Medical Emergency):

Immediate needle decompression is required without awaiting imaging.

Insert a 14- or 16-gauge needle with a catheter into the second intercostal space (ICS) at the midclavicular line.

Diagnosis is confirmed by the escape of high-pressure air.

2. Oxygen Therapy:

Administer supplemental oxygen while awaiting diagnostic confirmation.

Oxygen accelerates the reabsorption of air in the pleural space:

Normal absorption: ~1% per day.

100% oxygen therapy: Increases absorption to ~6% per day by replacing nitrogen in the pleural space with oxygen.

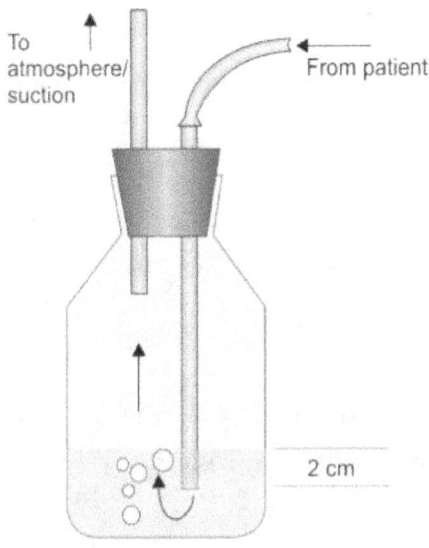

Fig. 9: Tube Thoracostomy with Underwater Seal

3. Tube Thoracostomy:

Recommended for secondary and traumatic pneumothorax.

Involves the placement of a chest tube to evacuate air from the pleural cavity.

4. Observation:

For primary spontaneous pneumothorax affecting <20% of the lung field without significant symptoms:

Monitoring is sufficient if serial CXRs at ~6 and 48 hours show no progression.

Keynote: Tension pneumothorax should always be diagnosed clinically due to its life-threatening nature. Immediate treatment with needle decompression takes precedence over confirmatory imaging.

Conclusion

Pneumothorax requires prompt identification and management tailored to its type and severity. Early intervention, particularly in emergencies like tension pneumothorax, significantly reduces mortality risk and improves outcomes.

Chapter 14
Hemoptysis

Introduction

Hemoptysis refers to the expectation of blood or blood-tinged sputum. Its severity is categorized as follows:

Mild: Blood loss of less than 100 mL per day.

Moderate: Blood loss of 100–150 mL per day.

Severe: Up to 200 mL per day.

Massive: Blood loss exceeding 500 mL daily, greater than 150 mL per hour, or more than 100 mL per day for over three days.

Massive hemoptysis, a life-threatening condition, typically arises from bleeding in the bronchial arteries in approximately 90% of cases. Common causes include bronchiectasis, bronchogenic carcinoma, tuberculosis, and fungal infections.

Differentiating hemoptysis from hematemesis is critical in emergency settings (refer to Table 1).

Hemoptysis vs. Hematemesis

Features	Hemoptysis	Haematemesis
Colour	Bright red	Dark brown or black
Consistency	Frothy, missed with sputum	Not frothy, mixed with food particles
Preceding symptom	Cough	Nausea or vomiting
Melena	Absent	Present
pH	Alkaline	Acidic

Medical history	Respiratory disease	Peptic ulcer or liver disease

Causes

1. Bronchiectasis: Chronic inflammation enlarges and distorts bronchial arteries near the affected airways.

2. Tuberculosis: Bleeding may result from bronchiolar ulceration, vascular necrosis, or rupture of a Rasmussen's aneurysm.

3. Fungal Infections: Includes aspergilloma, necrotizing pulmonary aspergillosis, histoplasmosis, and blastomycosis.

4. Bronchogenic Carcinoma: More common in centrally located squamous cell carcinomas.

5. Immunologic Lung Diseases: Goodpasture syndrome, Wegener's granulomatosis, systemic

lupus erythematosus (SLE), and microscopic polyangiitis.

6. Cardiac and Vascular Disorders: Pulmonary AV malformations, embolism, mitral stenosis, or aortic dissection.

Management

Airway Management

Hemoptysis can lead to airway obstruction and hypoxia due to alveolar flooding.

Administer supplemental oxygen to maintain $SpO_2 > 94\%$.

For massive hemoptysis: Insert a large-diameter endotracheal tube (≥8 mm) to allow bronchoscopy. If the source is identified, direct the tube to the unaffected lung to maintain ventilation.

Breathing

Position the patient with the bleeding lung in the dependent position (e.g., "lung down" approach) to protect the unaffected lung and enhance oxygenation.

Circulation

Massive bleeding may cause hemodynamic instability.

Establish IV access with a large-bore cannula.

Administer crystalloids and transfuse blood if necessary.

Correct coagulopathies.

Administer tranexamic acid: 1 g IV bolus, followed by 500 mg orally every 6 hours.

Antibiotics

Use antibiotics if there are signs of bacterial infection, such as in bronchitis or bronchiectasis.

Bronchoscopy

Early bronchoscopy aids in visualization and treatment, including:

Injection of vasoactive agents.

Balloon tamponade.

Topical hemostatic measures.

Thermocoagulation.

Imaging (CT Chest)

Perform a CT scan in stable patients to identify the bleeding site and guide potential interventions like embolization.

Interventional Angiography

Bronchial artery embolization (BAE): The first-line therapy for massive bleeding, particularly in cases due to tuberculosis or bronchiectasis.

Complications are rare but may include arterial dissection or perforation.

Summary

Hemoptysis management focuses on stabilizing the airway, addressing hemodynamic instability, and controlling the source of bleeding through imaging and interventional approaches. Early recognition and rapid interventions are crucial for favorable outcomes.

References

1. American Heart Association (AHA). (2020). Advanced Cardiovascular Life Support (ACLS) Provider Manual. American Heart Association.

2. Braunwald, E., Zipes, D. P., & Libby, P. (2019). Braunwald's Heart Disease: A Textbook of Cardiovascular Medicine (11th ed.). Elsevier.

3. Clement, R. (2019). Clinical Respiratory Medicine (5th ed.). Elsevier Health Sciences.

4. Holtzman, J. D., & Siegel, M. D. (2020). Cardiac Emergencies: Diagnosis and Management (2nd ed.). Springer.

5. Khera, A., & Vaduganathan, M. (2021). Cardiology: A Clinical Handbook. McGraw-Hill Education.

6. Liu, J., & Zhang, H. (2020). "Management of Acute Respiratory Distress Syndrome: Current Concepts and Therapies." Journal of Respiratory and Critical Care Medicine, 201(2), 12-29.

7. Long, B., & Koyfman, A. (2019). "Cardiac Emergencies in the Emergency Department." Emergency Medicine Clinics of North America, 37(4), 755-769.

8. National Heart, Lung, and Blood Institute (NHLBI). (2020). Acute Coronary Syndrome: Clinical Management and Diagnosis. NHLBI.

9. Squires, R. (2021). Respiratory Care: Principles and Practice (3rd ed.). Elsevier.

10. Thiele, H., & Werdan, K. (2018). Management of Acute Coronary Syndromes. Springer.

11. Tobin, M. J., & Jubran, A. (2020). "Management of Respiratory Failure and Acute

Respiratory Distress Syndrome." Textbook of Respiratory Medicine (2nd ed.). Elsevier.

12. Vincent, J. L., & Moreno, R. (2019). Critical Care Medicine: Principles of Diagnosis and Management in the Adult (5th ed.). Elsevier.

13. World Health Organization (WHO). (2021). Global Status Report on Cardiovascular Diseases. World Health Organization.

14. Zipes, D. P., & Libby, P. (2020). Cardiovascular Medicine (5th ed.). Elsevier.

www.ingramcontent.com/pod-product-compliance
Lightning Source LLC
Chambersburg PA
CBHW071028240526
45469CB00006BD/2138